Table of Contents

Introduction

An ulcer diet is intended to help reduce the pain and irritation that comes from a peptic ulcer—a painful sore that develops on the lining of your stomach, esophagus, or small intestine. Your doctor may put you on medication for your condition, but following an ulcer diet is an essential part of your overall care plan to manage symptoms and help your ulcer heal.

Foods or beverages don't cause ulcers, nor can they cure them. However, certain foods (e.g., fermented dairy foods) can help repair damaged tissue, and those that perpetuate acid build-up and inflammation (e.g., fried choices) may further aggravate your ulcer and threaten your digestive tract's natural layer of protection.

An ulcer diet is appropriate for anyone with an ulcer. It can also help those with gastritis or general stomach irritation.

Causes of Ulcers

There are many different causes of stomach ulcers. The most common among these are:

- **Helicobacter pylori infection.** Infection with the bacteria H. pylori can directly cause inflammation in the stomach and increase acid production. According to OMICS International, a consortium of journals and conference organizers, some 80% to 90% of stomach ulcers are caused by this bacterium.
- **NSAIDs.** Frequent or excessive use of nonsteroidal, anti-inflammatory drugs such as aspirin, ibuprofen and naproxen can impair the mucus lining of the stomach, leaving it susceptible to damage from stomach acid.
- **Tumors and other diseases.** Less common causes of ulcers include tumors that increase acid production in the stomach and stomach cancer, which can erode into the stomach, creating large ulcers.

No matter the cause of your stomach ulcers, healing them is important, not just to alleviate the pain and discomfort they can cause, but also for your long-term health. Left untreated, a stomach ulcer can turn into a serious problem. Complications may include:

- **Bleeding.** A broken blood vessel can cause bleeding into the stomach. This may show up as dark or bloody stools.
- **Obstruction.** Obstructions or blockages can develop that prevent food from moving through the digestive tract properly.
- **Perforations.** When the ulcer creates a hole in the stomach wall, this is called a perforation and is a very serious condition that allows digestive juices and food to leak into the abdominal cavity. This can lead to a potentially life-threatening infection.

- **Peritonitis.** This infection of the lining of the abdominal cavity can also become a serious issue.

Benefits of Ulcer Diet

Your doctor is far more likely to treat your ulcer with medications instead of diet alone, but adding an ulcer diet to your treatment can definitely help you feel better faster and possibly prevent another ulcer in the future.

Following an ulcer diet along with other treatment recommendations your doctor suggests can be beneficial because it can:

- Correct any nutritional deficiencies that may be contributing to your symptoms
- Provide the protein and other nutrients your body needs to heal

- Help you eliminate foods that aggravate the lining of your stomach or small intestine
- Help to control related conditions like Crohn's disease, celiac disease, or bacterial infections, which might be contributing to your ulcer

Most peptic ulcers are caused by long-term use of nonsteroidal anti-inflammatory drugs (NSAIDs), which can erode gastrointestinal lining, or by a bacterial infection known as Helicobacter pylori (H. pylori). An ulcer diet addresses both of these by including certain foods that have antibacterial properties and compounds that help promote healing.

How It Works

An ulcer diet works by helping to promote healing, avoiding irritation to the lining of your stomach or duodenum, and limiting excess acid production.

There are no strict rules about which foods to eat, but try to add as many foods as you can from the best choices list, and definitely avoid foods that make you feel worse or trigger excess acid production and reflux.

Eating enough protein is also important. While your ulcer is healing, aim for about 1.2 grams of protein per kilogram of your ideal body weight. The remainder of your calories should come from high fiber carbs like legumes, whole grains, fruits, and vegetables. A higher-fiber diet is associated with a lower risk of peptic ulcers. The report also advises adding some zinc and selenium to help with healing.

Duration

You should stay on an ulcer diet until your doctor tells you your ulcer is completely healed. Afterward, you can resume your normal way of eating. However, if you feel better while on the diet or you have risk factors for ulcers, like smoking, this way of eating may be worth continuing—even if in a modified way.

What to Eat and Avoid

Foods and Drinks to Avoid

While a generally healthy diet is considered best in supporting people with stomach ulcers, there tends to be a somewhat clearer list of foods to avoid. Although certain foods and beverages can cause stomach upset or increased production of stomach acid, there is no good evidence that they cause or worsen ulcers. Nevertheless, these foods may increase secretions of stomach acid, causing irritation of the stomach, or directly irritate the stomach wall.

Therefore, many people with stomach ulcers find that eating these foods makes them feel worse and thus they avoid them. Commonly avoided foods and beverages include:

- **Alcohol:** All alcohol is a stomach irritant and will delay healing. Avoid wine, beer, and spirits.

- **Caffeine:** You should cut back or eliminate coffee, tea, and caffeinated sodas, as these can increase stomach acid production.
- **Milk:** Milk used to be recommended as a treatment for ulcers, but the latest research has found that it increases stomach acid, so it's best to avoid it.
- **Certain meats:** Avoid highly-seasoned meats, lunch meats, sausages, and any fried or fatty meats and proteins.
- **High-fat foods:** Try to avoid large amounts of added fats, which can increase stomach acid and trigger reflux. You may need to avoid gravy, cream soups, and highly-seasoned salad dressings. (Healthy fats are OK.)
- **Spicy foods:** You may want to skip anything that is "hot" such as chili peppers, horseradish, black pepper, and sauces and condiments that contain them,

especially if they bother you or cause any pain or reflux.

- **Salty foods:** Researchers have found that highly salted foods may promote the growth of H. pylori.8 Be aware that pickles, olives, and other brined or fermented vegetables are high in salt and are associated with an increased risk of H. pylori ulcers.
- **Chocolate:** Chocolate can increase stomach acid production, and some people find that it triggers reflux symptoms.

Not everyone who has a stomach ulcer has problems with any or all of these foods, though. This is dependent on the person, so consider testing foods in small amounts or a short trial of elimination to see what irritates you.

Following an elimination diet for a while to determine exactly which foods cause you the most difficulty can help you dial in the right way of eating for you. Once you know what foods cause irritation (if any), continue to eat well-balanced, smaller and more frequent meals.

It's important that you continue to cover all your nutritional bases – eliminating certain foods could set you up for certain nutrient deficiencies if you're not including enough other foods that contain those nutrients. For example, make sure to include a protein-containing food at each meal.

You should seek to include legumes (beans, lentils) and healthy fats (avocado, olive oil) in your diet to provide good nutrition. And don't forget to drink plenty of water. Staying well hydrated has lots of health benefits and can promote better health of the digestive tract.

What to Eat If You Have Ulcers

A healthy, diversified diet rich in fruits, vegetables and fiber, and devoid of harmful artificial preservatives is key to helping your body heal its wounds. It's also important to avoid smoking cigarettes and drinking alcohol as these are risk factors for developing stomach ulcers.

Antioxidant properties of dietary polyphenols can support good gut health. (Polyphenols are compounds found in fruits and vegetables that support digestion and brain health and provide other health benefits.) Several items that are believed to be helpful in preventing or possibly even treating certain types of stomach ulcers, including:

- **Fruits:** Any fresh or frozen fruits are good and contribute beneficial fiber and antioxidants. Berries, apples, grapes, and pomegranates are among the best choices for ulcer healing polyphenols. If citrus fruits or juices like orange or grapefruit trigger reflux, avoid those.

- **Vegetables:** Leafy greens, bright red and orange vegetables, and cruciferous vegetables like broccoli, cauliflower, and kale are packed with vitamins and antioxidants that are especially good for your overall health and healing. Avoid spicy peppers and tomatoes/tomato products if they cause reflux. Limit raw vegetables, as they can be harder to digest.
- **Lean proteins:** Skinless poultry, lean beef like sirloin or tenderloin, fish, eggs, tofu, tempeh, dry beans, and peas are excellent sources of low-fat protein. Fatty fish like salmon, mackerel, and sardines provide omega-3 fats, which can reduce inflammation and may be helpful in preventing another ulcer.

- **Fermented dairy:** Products like kefir and Greek yogurt provide probiotics along with protein, so they're good choices.
- **Breads and grains:** 100% whole grain breads and whole or cracked grains like oats, quinoa, farro, millet, or sorghum are good sources of fiber to include in your diet.
- **Herbs and spices:** You can use most mild herbs and spices liberally. They're all concentrated sources of health-promoting antioxidants. Best bets include turmeric, cinnamon, ginger, and garlic, which have antimicrobial and anti-inflammatory properties. For a sweetener, try to use honey instead of sugar.

Recommended Timing

Try to eat five or six small meals each day, rather than three large ones. Stomach acid is produced every time you eat, but large meals require much more of it for digestion, which can be irritating. Finish up eating at least three hours before bedtime, and try to stay upright for a few hours after your last bite for improved digestion and less acid reflux.

Recipes to Help You Heal Ulcer

Carrot and Kale Quinoa Patties

Ingredients

- olive oil
- 1 1/2 cups cooked quinoa (equates to 1/2 cup uncooked quinoa)
- 2 tablespoons ground flaxseeds and 6 tablespoons of water, soaked for 10 minutes
- 1 cup kale, finely chopped (equates to approximately three leaves)
- 1/2 cup rolled oats, ground into flour (For a gluten-free patty, use gluten-free oats)
- 1/2 cup carrot, finely grated (equates to half of one large carrot)
- 1/4 cup pumpkin seeds
- 1/4 cup fresh basil, finely chopped

- 1/4 cup nutritional yeast
- 1/4 cup onion, finely diced
- equates to half a small onion
- 1 clove of garlic, minced
- 1 tablespoon tahini
- salt and pepper

Preparation

1. Preheat the oven to 400°F.
2. Line a baking tray with baking paper.
3. Heat the oil in a frying pan over a medium heat and cook the onions for five minutes or until soft. Add the garlic and cook for a further two minutes.
4. Combine all ingredients, including the cooked onion and garlic, together in a large bowl. Stir well until the mixture comes together.

5. With wet hands, shape mixture into 1/4 cup patties. Pack tightly so they will hold together better. Place onto lined baking tray.
6. Bake for 15 minutes then turn and bake for a further 10 minutes or until golden.
7. Allow to cool for 5 minutes then enjoy. Leftovers can be stored in the fridge to up to 5 days. Enjoy cold or to reheat, preheat a frying pan, and cook patties for about 3 minutes on each side in a little bit of oil.

Matcha Berry Pancakes

Ingredients

For the Wet Mix:

- 1 tablespoon flax seeds, ground
- 2 1/2 tablespoons warm water
- 2/3 cup almond milk, unsweetened
- 1 teaspoon vanilla extract
- 1 teaspoon apple cider vinegar
- 1 tablespoon olive oil

For the Dry Mix:

- 1 cup gluten free all-purpose flour
- 1 teaspoon baking powder
- 1/4 teaspoon baking soda
- 1/4 teaspoon salt
- 1 teaspoon matcha powder

For the Pancake Garnish:

- Berries
- Maple syrup
- Vegan butter

Preparation

1. For the wet mix, in a bowl mix the ground flax and the warm water and allow to sit for 10 minutes.
2. Add the almond milk, vanilla extract, apple cider vinegar and olive oil and stir well. Set aside until ready to add to the dry mix.
3. For the dry mix, add the flour, baking powder, baking soda, salt and matcha to a bowl and whisk till well mixed. Add the wet mix and stir until most of the lumps are gone. Be careful not to over stir!
4. To cook the pancakes, heat a skillet over medium heat and add a small amount of oil to the pan. Ladle out a portion of the pancake batter into the pan.

5. Sprinkle some of the fresh fruit around the top of the pancake.
6. Cook until the pancake is bubbling around the edges and then flip (after about 4 minutes).
7. Cook on the other side about 4-5 minutes or until cooked all the way through.
8. To serve, top with more berries, maple syrup and vegan butter!

Baked Broccoli Burgers

Ingredients

For the Burgers:

- 1/3 cup dry couscous
- 1 cup water
- 1 1/2 cups broccoli florets
- 2 teaspoons olive oil
- 1/2 cup chopped scallions
- 1/2 cup chopped yellow onion
- 2 teaspoons ground cumin
- 1 15-ounce can of chickpeas, rinsed and drained
- 1 tablespoon tahini
- 1/2 cup panko bread crumbs

For the Tahini Dressing:

- 1/3 cup tahini
- 1/3 cup water

- 1/4 cup, plus 1 tablespoon fresh lemon juice
- 2 garlic cloves, chopped
- 3/4 teaspoon sea salt

Preparation

1. Preheat your oven to 400°F.
2. In a small pot, bring the water and couscous to a boil.
3. Remove from heat immediately and allow the couscous to sit in the pot for 10 minutes, soaking up the water.
4. While the couscous sits, steam the broccoli in a steamer for 5-7 minutes (or use a microwave or stove method, you just want the broccoli to be soft in the end).
5. In a skillet, heat the olive oil over medium heat and add the onion and scallions, stirring occasionally for 3-5 minutes until the onion softens.
6. Remove the onions from the heat and stir in the cumin.

7. Gather your couscous, broccoli, onion mix, chickpeas, and tahini and combine together in a food processor.
8. Pour the mixture into a bowl and stir in the bread crumbs.
9. Form it into patties and place the patties on a cookie sheet lined with foil.
10. Bake for 50 minutes, turning the patties over halfway through. You'll know they are done when the tops begin to brown.
11. To make the tahini sauce, place all ingredients in a food processor and blend until combined, roughly 30 seconds.
12. Top your burgers with the sauce, throw some pickles, tomato, and lettuce on top, and serve.

Instant Pot Cabbage Soup

Ingredients

- 2 tablespoons olive oil
- 1 cup carrots
- 1 cup celery
- 1/2 cup yellow onion
- 1 teaspoon sea salt
- 1/2 teaspoon black pepper
- 1 teaspoon Italian herb seasoning
- 3 cloves garlic, minced
- 4 cups cabbage, shredded
- 1 cup sweet corn
- 1 cup zucchini
- 4 cups vegetable broth

Preparation

1. Add oil to the instant pot and turn it on the sauté function. Add carrots, celery, and onion and sauté 5 minutes until softened.
2. Add garlic and sauté 3 more minutes.
3. Add cabbage, corn, zucchini, and broth, then stir to combine. Set the instant pot to soup function for 20 minutes. After 20 minutes, turn the valve to instant release. After pressure has released, open and stir. Serve and enjoy!

Lychee and Kombucha Spritz

Ingredients

- 12 lychees, peeled and seeds removed
- 10 sprigs of mint
- 1/2 lime
- 2 cups kombucha of your choice (choose one with little additional sweetener if you can)
- 10 ice cubes

Preparation

1. Add slices of lime, 5 sprigs of mint, and 5 ice cubes to each glass or jar.
2. Add 5 peeled and seeded lychees to each glass/jar.
3. Pour 1/2 of kombucha into each glass/jar and stir ingredients together well.
4. Garnish with a fresh lychee and mint.

Cafe Style Matcha Tea Latte

Ingredients

- 1 teaspoon matcha
- 2 oz water
- 6-10 oz nut milk
- 1 teaspoon vanilla extract
- 1 teaspoon agave
- Cacao powder or matcha to sprinkle

Preparation

1. Place 1 teaspoon Matcha into a cup.
2. Melt Matcha by adding 2 oz hot water and stirring until matcha becomes a smooth paste.
3. Add vanilla and agave to milk and warm.
4. Pour 6-10 oz steamed milk into Matcha tea.
5. Scoop foamy milk on top.
6. Sprinkle with Matcha dust or cacao powder.

Fresh Cranberry Scones

Ingredients

- 1 package fresh cranberries, minimum 6 ounces, maximum 12 ounces
- 1/3 cup brown sugar, not packed
- 2 1/4 cups AP flour
- 3 teaspoons baking powder
- 1/2 teaspoon salt
- zest of 2 organic oranges
- 1/4 chopped candied ginger
- 10 tablespoons chilled coconut oil, cut into small pieces
- 1/3 soy/almond milk

Preparation

1. Preheat oven 350ºF and line baking sheet with parchment paper.

2. In food processor, pulse the cranberries with the brown sugar and orange zest. Go for chunky. Put in large mixing bowl, set aside.
3. In food processor, pulse the AP flower, baking powder and salt.
4. Add in the coconut oil and pulse until pea-sized crumbles appear.
5. Mix the flour mixture with the cranberries in the mixing bowl.
6. Add the milk and stir until it just comes together.
7. Dust counter with a bit of flour, dump dough onto it. Form a disk/thick circle.
8. Cut into quarters, and within those quarters cut 3 wedges.
9. Carefully transfer wedges on prepared baking sheet and bake for 40-45 minutes, rotating the baking sheet half way through.

10. The edges and bottom will darken a little, but the interior will be tender and crumbly.
11. Serve warm, as is, or drizzled with icing (you can make a quick icing slurry of 2 teaspoons the milk used + enough powdered sugar to get a thickened but drizzly consistency, anywhere from 10-15 tablespoons).

Cocoa Brownies

Ingredients

- 1/2 cup flour or 1/2 cup ground almonds
- 1/2 tsp salt (kosher)
- 1 1/4 cup unsweatened Cocoa powder
- 1 cup Granulated Sugar
- 1 cup Brown Sugar (packed)
- 1 tbsp Vanilla extract
- 1 cup Light Margarine (softened)
- 1 large egg
- 3 egg whites from large eggs
- 1/2 tsp cinnamon
- (1/8 tsp cyanne pepper optional)

Directions

1. Preheat oven to 300 degrees. Grease a 9x13 pan with non-stick spray. (you can use butter, but why add the calories).
2. Cream the margarine and sugars. Then add the other wet ingredients.
3. Sift together the cocoa powder and flour/almonds. You can use either flour or almonds- the difference in calories is minimal(almonds is a trace more).
4. Add the cinnamon and optional cyanne pepper.
5. It's handy to have a kitchen-aid mixer or other stand mixer at this point, but a hand held is also ok.
6. Use the paddle attachment. Beat to combine for about 20-30 seconds- wipe down sides. Then mix at medium speed for 4 minutes. Batter will be very wet.
7. Pour in to your prepared pan and bake at 300 for about 45 minutes.

8. Toothpick test in the center to see if done. Brownies will be very moist- that's what makes them irresistable!

**To make these diabetic friends, you can replace the sugars with spelda white & brown sugars- just follow the conversions provided on the package. Good for diabetics and carb friendly. You can also switch to promise or earth balance butter sticks.

Vegetarian Gumbo

Ingredients

- 1 onion, chopped
- 1 c celery, diced
- 4 garlic cloves, minced
- 2 teaspoons dried thyme (or 2 tablespoons fresh thyme, minced)
- 1 bay leaf
- 1 (28 ounce) can diced tomatoes
- 1/2 uncooked cup rice
- 4 cups vegetable broth
- 2 teaspoons paprika
- 4 teaspoons lemon juice
- salt (optional)
- 2 cups okra, sliced (I use frozen)
- 1 green pepper, diced
- 1 -2 dash hot pepper sauce (Tabasco)

Directions

1. Saute onions and celery until transparent in large frying pan. If you use oil for this (I just use a little spray), then you need to add it to the nutrition calculations. Add minced garlic. Saute another minute.
2. Add tomatoes, bring to boil from 1-2 minutes.
3. Transfer to large crock pot. Add rice and broth.
4. Cook on low for 6 hours - until rice is tender (OR cook on high 3 hours)
5. Mix paprika and lemon juice in small bowl. Add lemon, paprika, okra, and diced peppers to crock pot. Cook on high for 20 minutes until heated throughout.
6. Serve and enjoy!

Mexican Black Bean Salad

Ingredients

- 1 1/2 cups cooked black beans
- 3 scallions (green onions) sliced
- 2 ripe plum tomatoes, diced
- 1/3 cup corn, fresh, frozen or canned
- 2 tablespoons olive oil
- 1 tablespoon fresh lime juice
- 2 tablespoons freshly chopped cilantro
- salt and freshly ground black pepper to taste
- minced garlic and/or hot peppers may be added for an extra zesty flavor

Directions

1. Combine all ingredients in a medium size bowl and toss gently. Let the salad rest in the refrigerator until serving time.

2. Use this simple recipe as a starting point. Add green or red pepper, parsley, etc. to personalize this salad.

Coconut Dream Pie

Ingredients

- 2 envelopes Kraft Dream Whip Topping - dry mix (unprepared)
- 2 3/4 cup skim milk
- 1 tsp vanilla extract
- 1 tsp coconut extract (optional)
- 2 (4 serving) boxes fat-free vanilla pudding mix
- 1 cup coconut, toasted
- 1 (9-inch) graham cracker crust (may use any type shell you wish, or serve this as a mousse without a shell)

Directions

- Beat whipped topping mix, 1 cup of milk and vanilla on high for 6 minutes till very stiff (6 minutes ... don't under beat)
- Add remaining milk and pudding mixes, and coconut extract (if using) beat on high for 2 minutes. Fold in coconut, pour into pie shell.
- Reserve 2 TBSP of coconut for garnish if desired.
- Chill at least 4 hrs. Sprinkle with reserved coconut or a few very fine chocolate curls to garnish.

Note: To save almost 100 calories per serving ... do not make in a pie shell. Instead, fill individual dessert cups with pie filling and sprinkle ligtly with low fat graham cracker crumbs (toasted).

Flourless Tiny Peanut Butter Cookies

Ingredients

- 1 cup unsalted natural peanut butter
- 1/2 cup Splenda brown sugar (packed)
- 1/4 cup egg substitute (such as Egg Beaters brand)
- 1/2 tsp vanilla extract
- 40 pieces semisweet chocolate chips or semisweet chocolate candies

Directions

1. Preheat oven to 350 degrees F.
2. Lightly spray a cookie sheet with canola oil.
3. In a medium size mixing bowl, place the peanut butter, brown sugar, egg substitute, and vanilla extract. Stir together well.

4. Using a small scoop, equal to about a rounded measuring teaspoon, drop cookie dough on the prepared cookie sheet.
5. Take a fork and make a criss-cross pattern on each cookie.
6. Add one mini chocolate chip or mini chocolate candy to the top of each cookie.
7. Bake approximately 8 or 9 minutes or until cookie is lightly browned on bottom.
8. Remove cookie sheet from oven and let rest on a cooling rack for 5 minutes before removing cookies to rack to continue cooling.
9. Makes approximately 40 tiny cookies. YUMMY!

Nutritional Info: Servings Per Recipe: 40

Amount Per Serving Calories: 57.7 Total Fat: 3.9 g Cholesterol: 0.2 mg Sodium: 35.1 mg Total Carbs: 3.6 g Dietary Fiber: 0.2 g Protein: 2.2 g

Spaghetti Sauce with Ground Turkey

Minutes to Prepare: 10 Minutes to Cook: 20 Number of Servings: 8

Ingredients

- *Extra Virgin Olive Oil, 2 tbsp
- Garlic, 4 cloves
- Onions, raw, 1 cup, chopped
- Turkey, Ground turkey, 93% lean, 16 oz
- Oregano, ground, 3 tbsp
- Basil, 2 tbsp
- Bay leaf, whole (remove before serving)
- Parsley, dried, 1 tbsp
- Tomato Sauce, no salt added, 2 cup

Directions

1. heat onion and minced garlic in extra virgin olive oil until onions are nearly translucent.

2. add ground turkey to pan cover with seasoning and brown
3. add tomato sauce and heat thoroughly.
4. Serve over gluten free pasta.
5. I often add more italian seasoning, or more tomato sauce or paste. It just depends on taste.

Nutritional Info: Amount Per Serving Calories: 156.5 Total Fat: 7.7 g Cholesterol: 0.0 mg Sodium: 74.6 mg Total Carbs: 11.6 g Dietary Fiber: 3.2 g Protein: 13.6 g

Low Carb/Sugar Free/Gluten Free/Almond Cookies

Minutes to Prepare: 15 Minutes to Cook: 20 Number of Servings: 12

Ingredients

- 1 stick softened butter
- 2 cups almond flour
- 1/2 cup splenda
- 1 tsp vanilla extract
- 1 tsp almond extrack
- 12 whole almonds

Directions

1. preheat oven 300 deg
2. soften 1 stick butter
3. add 2c almond flour & 1/2c splenda
4. & mix well with a fork

5. add vanilla & almond extract & continue to mix
6. roll into walnut size balls & place on lightly oiled cookie sheet
7. place in oven for 5 min
8. remove & press down with fork in a cris cross fashion & place a whole almond in center
9. return to oven for an additional 15 to 17 min
10. remove from oven & allow to cool before transfering to a rack
11. enjoy

Nutritional Info Servings Per Recipe: 12

Amount Per Serving Calories: 103.1 Total Fat: 10.6 g Cholesterol: 20.3 mg Sodium: 54.5 mg Total Carbs: 2.5 g Dietary Fiber: 0.6 g Protein: 1.3 g

Pumpkin Muffin in a Cup

Minutes to Prepare: 2 Minutes to Cook: 1 Number of Servings: 1

Ingredients

- 1 large Egg, fresh, whole, raw
- 0.50 tsp Cinnamon, ground
- 0.25 tsp Nutmeg, ground
- 0.50 tsp Pumpkin Pie spice
- 0.50 tsp Baking Powder
- 1/4 Cup Flax Seed Meal (ground flax)
- 3 Tbs Libby's 100% pure canned pumpkin
- 1.5 tsp Truvia Baking Blend Natural Sweetener with Sugar - serving size 1/2 tsp (2g)

Tips

Add cream cheese and honey icing at your own risk - sparingly.

Directions

1. Mix all together in a mug and microwave for 1 min 40 sec!

Nutritional Info: Amount Per Serving Calories: 257.0 Total Fat: 14.4 g Cholesterol: 186.0 mg Sodium: 318.1 mg Total Carbs: 21.3 g Dietary Fiber: 11.4 g Protein: 13.4 g

Keto 90 second bread

Minutes to Prepare: 1 Minutes to Cook: 1 Number of Servings: 2

Ingredients

- 1 tbsp Coconut flour
- 1/4 cup Bob's Red Mill Almond Meal/Flour
- 1 large Egg, fresh, whole, raw
- 1/4 tsp Baking Powder
- 1 tsp Coconut Oil

Tips

You can use this bread anytime not just for breakfast. Takes 30 seconds to prep and 90 seconds to cook.

Directions

1. Place all ingredients in mug or ramekin, mix well to combine. Cook in microwave for 90 seconds. Remove and run a butter knife around outer side of mug then turn over onto plate (sometimes it will come out on its own) slice horizontally into two slices.

Nutritional Info: Amount Per Serving Calories: 166.7 Total Fat: 12.7 g Cholesterol: 93.0 mg Sodium: 96.5 mg Total Carbs: 7.4 g Dietary Fiber: 3.0 g Protein: 7.2 g

Flour-less Brownies with Splenda

Minutes to Prepare: 15 Minutes to Cook: 30 Number of Servings: 35

Ingredients

- 1 cup Splenda (can do half splenda half regular sugar... which will be a little more cals)
- 1/2 cup Almonds (ground)
- 1/4 cup Splenda Brown Sugar
- 2 sticks Butter Unsalted
- 3 Egg Whites
- 1 Large Egg
- 1 cup Cocoa Powder (unsweetened)
- 2 dashes of Cinnamon (1/2-1 tsp)

Directions

1. Preheat oven to 300 degrees.
2. Grease a 9x13 pan with non-stick spray.

3. Combine butter and sugars and wet ingredients in a bowl (medium)
4. Mix cocoa powder and ground almonds in a separate bowl then combine to wet ingredients
5. Add the cinnamon. * Batter will be very wet...
6. Pour in to your prepared pan and bake at 300 degrees for about 30 minutes until your toothpick or fork comes out clean in the middle Brownies will be very moist but and delicious!

Nutritional Info: Amount Per Serving Calories: 81.9 Total Fat: 7.4 g Cholesterol: 11.8 mg Sodium: 71.4 mg Total Carbs: 4.3 g Dietary Fiber: 1.2 g Protein: 1.7 g

Simple Peanut butter brownies

Minutes to Prepare: 5 Minutes to Cook: 22 Number of Servings: 9

Ingredients

- 1 cup natural peanut butter (works with any kind tho)
- 1/2 cup honey
- 1 egg
- 1/2 tsp baking soda

Directions

1. Mix all ingredients with a handmixer until smooth
2. pour into 8X8 brownie pan
3. bake at 350 for 22 to 25 minutes

Nutritional Info: Amount Per Serving Calories: 220.4 Total Fat: 15.2 g Cholesterol: 23.6 mg Sodium: 280.7 mg Total Carbs: 17.1 g Dietary Fiber: 1.7 g

Easy Peanutbutter Cookies

Minutes to Prepare: 10 Minutes to Cook: 10 Number of Servings: 24

Ingredients

- 1C Peanutbutter (we like Jif)
- 1C Sugar (optional: 1/2c more)
- 1 egg

Directions

1. Mix thoroughly. Make small balls of dough (smaller than a golf ball) then roll it is a plate of sugar to coat ball (optional). Place on pan and smoosh with fork twice, making hatch marks. Cook 350 degrees 7-10 min. Recipe does not include the sugar coating - if you skip it no one will know.

Nutritional Info: Amount Per Serving Calories: 98.6 Total Fat: 5.5 g Cholesterol: 8.9 mg Sodium: 52.6 mg Total Carbs: 10.7 g Dietary Fiber: 0.7 g Protein: 2.9 g

Peanut butter truffle cookies

Minutes to Prepare: 10 Minutes to Cook: 10 Number of Servings: 24

Ingredients

- 1 cup creamy peanut butter (I like all natural Skippy)
- 1 cup brown sugar, firmly packed
- 1 large egg
- 1 teaspoon baking soda
- 1/2 cup semi-sweet chocolate chips

Directions

1. Preheat oven to 350.

2. Combine all ingredients except chips until well blended (seriously, my cookies still had some sugar graininess).
3. Add chips.
4. Drop slightly rounded teaspoonfulls on ungreased cookie sheets (12 to a sheet) - do not flatten.
5. Bake 10 minutes or until puffed and golden. Cool on wire rack for at least 5 minutes before removing from cookie sheet (they will be very soft).

Makes 24 - 30 cookies

Nutritional Info: Amount Per Serving Calories: 124.3 Total Fat: 6.6 g Cholesterol: 8.9 mg Sodium: 59.0 mg Total Carbs: 13.2 g Dietary Fiber: 0.9 g Protein:

Four Cheese Macaroni and Cheese

Minutes to Prepare: 30 Minutes to Cook: 15 Number of Servings: 5

Ingredients

Sauce:

- 2 tbsp butter
- 2 tbsp Namaste Gluten Free Flour Blend
- 2 cups skim milk
- 1 bay leaf
- 1/2 cup onion
- 3/4 cup reduce fat mexican style blend cheese (reserve 1/4 cup) for the topping)
- 1/4 tsp salt
- 1 tsp yellow mustard (the kind in the squeeze bottle. Make sure it says "gluten free".)
- 8 ounces Deboles gluten free elbow corn pasta

- 6 slices turkey bacon, cooked and chopped

Directions

1. Preheat oven to 375 degrees. Prepare a 9" x 13" casserole dish and coat it with either non stick spray, or Spectrum non hydrogenated shortening.
2. Put butter in a medium sauce pan and heat it until it comes to a bubble add in the chopped onion and let cook for a minute.
3. Whisk in flour, milk, salt, pepper, paprika, and mustard.
4. Add in a whole bay leaf and the parsley.
5. Let the mixture warm over medium heat and stir frequently to prevent burning. Add in a 1/2 cup of the cheese and TURN OFF the heat. Set mixture aside.
6. Cook the pasta according to package directions in salted water.
7. Steam or microwave 3 cups of broccoli pieces.

8. Chopp up turkey bacon and crisp slightly in frying pan.
9. Drain pasta when it is finished cooking and pour it into the casserole dish.
10. Pour the broccoli in with the pasta and stir around.
11. Remove the bay leaf from the cheese mixture and throw away.
12. Pour cheese mixture over pasta and broccoli and mix well.
13. Top with remaining cheese and bake in the oven for 15 minutes.
14. Enjoy!

Nutritional Info: Calories: 370.0 Total Fat: 12.4 g Cholesterol: 41.1 mg Sodium: 585.3 mg Total Carbs: 52.6 g Dietary Fiber: 7.7 g Protein: 15.2 g

Cioppino

Ingredients

- 100g fish or seafood of choice
- 1 chopped tomato
- 2 c broth
- 2-3 cloves minced garlic
- 1 bay leaf
- 1 t dehydrated minced onion
- 1 t parsley
- 1/4 t oregano
- 1/4 t basil
- 1/8 t rosemary
- 1/8 t fennel seeds
- salt/pepper to taste
- tabasco

Directions

1. Combine minced onion, parsley, oregano, basil, rosemary, and fennel seeds in food processor or grinder. Grind.
2. Add seasonings and all other ingredients except for seafood & tabasco in saucepan.
3. Bring to a boil. Reduce heat, cover, and simmer for 30 mins.
4. Add fish and return to boil.
5. Reduce heat, cover, and simmer 5-15 mins.
6. Remove bay leaf.
7. Top with a few dashes of tabasco just before serving.

NOTE: For the tomato on this dish, I will sometimes chop up a few slices of tomato and then add 2 T of sugar free natural tomato sauce for a slightly more tomatoey taste.

Muffin in a Minute

Ingredients

- 1/4 cup flax meal (8.09 total carbs, 7.6 fiber)
- 1/2 teaspoon baking powder (0.64 net carbs)
- 1 packet splenda packet (0.9 net carbs)
- 1 teaspoon cinnamon (1.84 total carbs, 1.2 fiber)
- 1 large egg (0.6 net carbs)
- 1 teaspoon butter

Directions

1. Put the dry ingredients in a coffee mug.
2. Stir.
3. Then add the egg and the butter. Mix.
4. Microwave 1 minute (or more). Take out. slice, butter, enjoy.
5. Cream cheese would go nicely, too.

6. The shape of this can be changed by making it in a bowl.
7. It can be "toasted" once it's cooked.
8. The cinnamon can be replaced. I would imagine that any sugar free syrup could be added.
9. Some people count the flax as a carb/fiber wash, so then the net carbs would be 2.78.

Dark Chocolate Coconut Fat Bombs

Ingredients

1. 0.65 cup Organics unsweetened shedded coconut
2. 8 pieces baking chocolate
3. 20 gram Sam's choice swiss dark chocolate
4. 5 tbsp Kirkland Organic Virgin Coconut Oil Serving Size 1 tbsp (14g)
5. 3 serving Truvia Natural Sweetener

Directions

1. Melt ingredients add coconut divide into 10 portions

   Serving Size: 1

Bowl of Cheesecake

Ingredients

- 2 oz 1/3 less fat Philly cream cheese
- 1 tbsp sour cream
- 2 pkts Equal (or Splenda)

Directions

1. Soften cream cheese in microwave for 30 seconds or less, stir in sour cream and sweetener, enjoy warm or chill.
2. Stir in s/t flavorings as desired.

Flax Pancakes

Ingredients

- 1 egg
- 3 T. flax seed meal
- 1/2 t. baking powder
- 1/2 t. vanilla
- 1-2 packets splenda
- cinnamon and/or nutmeg to taste

Directions

1. Heat a skillet to medium heat.
2. Spray with PAM or similar.
3. Mix everything together and pour onto skillet.
4. Basically cook like a normal pancake.
5. You can top with sugar-free pancake syrup or SB friendly margarine like smart balance, if desired.

Refried Bean Soup

Ingredients

- 1 16 oz. can Fat Free Refried Beans*
- 1 cup Canned Yellow Corn
- 1 16 oz. can Chicken Broth*
- 1 16 oz. can Ro-tel Original Tomatoes w/ Green Chilies
- 1 cup Canned Black Beans (drained)
- 8 Tbsp Fat Free Sour Cream

Directions

1. Mix everything (except sour cream) together into a pot and simmer until heated through, whisking to combined refried beans with the chicken broth.
2. Serve 1 cup servings in bowls and top each with 2 tbsp of Sour Cream.

*Use vegatarian refried beans and vegetable stock to make this soup vegetarian friendly.

Baked Kale Chips

Ingredients

- 1 Bunch Kale
- Nutritional Yeast
- Spices

Preparation

1. Preheat oven or toaster oven to 225F.
2. Tear kale into uniform-sized pieces, but don't make the pieces too small – they will shrink down.
3. Place kale on a non-stick cookie sheet or a cookie sheet lined with parchment paper.
4. Sprinkle generously with spices such as nutritional yeast, Old Bay seasoning, sea salt, garlic salt or anything you like.
5. Bake for 7-10 minutes until the kale pieces are dark green and crispy, taking care not to burn them.

Simple Peanut butter brownies

Ingredients

- 1 cup natural peanut butter (works with any kind tho)
- 1/2 cup honey
- 1 egg
- 1/2 tsp baking soda

Directions

1. Mix all ingredients with a handmixer until smooth
2. pour into 8X8 brownie pan
3. bake at 350 for 22 to 25 minutes

Cheesy Chicken, Broccoli and Rice Casserole

Ingredients

- 2 cups cooked shredded chicken
- 4 cups instant white rice
- 4 cups chicken broth
- 1 bag frozen chopped broccoli
- 16 oz Light 2% Velveeta Cheese (1/2 big block)
- 1 can cream of mushroom soup

Directions

1. Preheat oven to 350 degrees. Cook broccoli on stove or steam in microwave.
2. Boil chicken broth, add rice, remove from heat covered.
3. Let stand 5 minutes or until broth is completely absorbed.

4. While rice is standing, chop velveeta into blocks so melting is easier.
5. Combine shredded chicken, velveeta and cream of mushroom soup.
6. Add cooked broccoli and rice and mix thoroughly.
7. Transfer to casserole dish and bake at 350 degrees for 20-30 minutes.

1 serving = 1 cup. 1 cup = 5 weight watcher points

Homemade "Atkins" Shake

Ingredients

- 2 eggs
- 1 T virgin coconut oil
- 1 T butter
- 1 T cocoa powder or Instant decaf coffee
- 1/4 t cinnamon
- 1/4 t pumpkin pie spice
- stevia to taste (optional)
- boiling water 4-6 oz
- ice cubes

Directions

1. Break 2 eggs into blender. Add all ingredients except ice.
2. Blend. Add ice to desired consistency. Enjoy!

Note: Don't shy away from this because of the "raw eggs" The boiling water cooks them just enough & then everything is blended. I don't like slimy things and I LOVE this shake!

I brew a pot of good french roast coffee and then keep it in the refrigerator. I boil some in the microwave and this is my "boiling water", instead.

Cranberry Waldorf Salad

Ingredients

- 1 1/2 cup Oceanspray Craisins (any flavor)
- 1/2 Cup Raisins
- 1/2 cup Chopped Red Apple
- 1/2 cup Chopped Green Apple
- 1 Cup Chopped Celery
- 1 Cup Seedless Red Grapes
- 1/2 Cup Chopped Walnuts

- 3 TBS. Fat Free Miracle Whip

SUBSTITUTIONS:

- Substitute the Miracle Whip for 8 oz. of low fat Plain Vanilla Yogurt
- Substitute Walnuts for Pecans

ADDITIONS:

- Mini-Marshmallows are delicious in this recipe if you don't mind a few added calories or want to make a kid-friendly version.

Directions

1. Toss all ingredients into a large bowl making sure to stir in the Miracle Whip or yogurt well.
2. Cover and chill for 2 hours before serving.

Veggie Joes

Ingredients

- Garlic, 2 cloves, minced
- 1 Onion, chopped
- 1/4 c Banana Peppers
- 2C TVP, reconstituted with 1 3/4 c water 12 oz Tomato Sauce
- 1 tsp Oregano
- 1/4 c Catsup
- 2T Worcestershire Sauce (vegan friendly brand)
- 2 T Brown Sugar

Directions

1. Saute first 4 ingredients in a large frying pan.
2. In a bowl combine remaining ingredients. Stir into frying pan and bring to a boil.
3. Add salt and pepper to taste.

4. Reduce heat and stir until sauce is thickened.
5. Serve over bread of choice and enjoy!

Mini Cheesy Meatloaves

Ingredients

- 8 oz extra lean ground beef
- 1 small egg
- 1/2 cup chopped fresh onion
- 1/2 cup rolled quick oats (dry)
- 4 tbsp ketchup
- 2 tsp yellow mustard
- 2 tbsp brown sugar barbeque sauce
- 1 oz marbled cheddar cheese (cubed into 6 tiny cubes)

Directions

1. Preheat oven to 375.

2. In medium mixing bowl, add all ingredients EXCEPT for cheese. Mix well.
3. Drop beef mixture by spoonfuls into 6 ungreased, unlined muffin tins.
4. Place 1 small cube of cheese into center of each mini-meatloaf. Press down.
5. Bake in oven for 30 minutes.
6. Serves 6.

Christmas Punch

Ingredients

- 64 oz 100% Cranberry juice
- 2 liter Diet Sprite Zero
- 1 cup Cranberrie,s optional
- 2 limes
- ice

Directions

1. Pour cranberry juice and sprite into punch bowl.
2. Then chop cranberries and slice limes. Add fruit to punch.
3. Cover and chill.
4. Add ice when ready to serve.

No Bake Chocolate Coconut Cookies

Ingredients

- 3 c. oatmeal, instant or old fashioned (chewier)
- 1 c. coconut, shredded
- 1/4 c. cocoa, (Hershey's special dark make the best cookies)
- 1/2 c. butter
- 1/2 c. milk
- 2 c. sugar
- 1 t. vanilla

Directions

1. In a medium bowl mix oatmeal, coconut and cocoa.
2. In a medium saucepan melt butter, add milk, sugar and vanilla.
3. Bring to a full boil. Boil for 2 minutes.
4. Remove from heat and pour over oatmeal mixture.

5. Stir until well combined. Spoon onto wax paper to cool. Makes about 25 cookies.

Easy Baked Chicken

Ingredients

- 1lb of skinless chicken breasts cut into thin strips (or you can leave in big pieces if you like, but kids like the strips better)
- 1-2 tbsp of olive oil (or i like to use the olive oil cooking spray, its so easy)
- 1/2 cup of italian bread crumbs
- 1/2 cup of shredded parmesean
- 2 tbsp of minced garlic

Directions

1. Preheat oven to 375. Spray an oven safe dish with cooking spray.

2. Mix breadcrumbs, garlic and parmesean in small bowl. Rub olive oil (or spray on) both sides of each piece of chicken.
3. Then dredge each piece of chicken in breadcrumb mixture and plae in oven dish.
4. Place dish in oven for 20-30min or until cooked through.
5. Enjoy!

Bleu Cheese Salad Dressing

Ingredients

- 2 cups mayo
- 2 cups souor cream
- 1 tsp Worchestershire sauce
- 2 cloves garlic minced
- 2 shallots minced
- 1/3 cup balsamic Vinegar
- 1 cup or more, whatever your taste is bleu cheese
- 1 tbsp NSA applesauce

Directions

1. Mix the first 3 ingredients together
2. Take the minced garlic and shallots and put them in a small saucepan with the balsamic vinegar.

3. Reduce the vinegar by 1/2. It will become thick like syrup. It will also stink up the house, but it will go away. This is such an important step.
4. Add the reduction to the first three ingredients.
5. Wait of course, until it cools off.
6. Add the bleu cheese and the applesauce.
7. Mix well, cover and let it all marinate for about 2 hrs. Then enjoy.
8. I don't add salt, but you may want to. Also a little pepper if you want.

Salmon Cakes

INGREDIENTS

- 2 (7 ounce) can salmon, drained, deboned, and flaked
- 1 egg, beaten
- 1 tablespoon olive oil
- 1 onion, finely chopped
- 1/2 cup instant potatoes (do not add milk,etc)
- Salt and pepper to taste (or you can use Old Bay Seasoning if you have it)

Directions

1. Preheat oven to 375 degrees. Spray cookie sheet well with cooking spray.
2. Mix all the ingredients together and shape into patties.
3. Place on well sprayed cookie sheet, and bake for 20 minutes turning once.

(Note: You can fry these also, which is what my Grandfather use to do, but you will save calories if you bake them.)

Huevo Ranchero

Ingredients

- 1/2 cup black beans (or fat-free refried black beans)
- dash cumin, if desired
- 1/2 thin slice red onion
- 1/2 oz. shredded reduced-fat cheese
- 1 egg
- 2 Tbsp. sugar-free salsa
- 2 Tbsp. guacamole (homemade without out salt, will reduce sodium)

Directions

1. Poach egg in simmering water.

2. While egg is poaching, put beans in a microwave-safe bowl, and mash slightly with a dash of cumin, if desired.
3. Top with onion and cheese, and microwave for about 30-45 seconds, until cheese is melted.
4. Top with egg and then salsa, and put guacamole on side.

The Bottomline

If you have any type of stomach pain, nausea, vomiting or any other gastrointestinal symptoms that last longer than a few days, always consult your doctor. Ulcers can be serious if they cause internal bleeding. An ulcer diet is meant to help, but your doctor should be aware of your efforts and recommend a comprehensive treatment plan.

BBQ Chicken Pizza

Ingredients

- 1 - 10 oz whole wheat pizza crust
- 8 oz cooked boneless, skinless chicken breast, diced
- 3/4 cup BBQ sauce
- 1/2 cup low fat shredded cheddar cheese
- 1/4 cup diced red onion

Directions

1. Spread BBQ sauce on pizza
2. Top with diced chicken, cheese, & red onion.
3. Cook on 450 degrees for 8 - 10 minutes

Skinny Pina' Colada

Ingredients

- 1 1/2 oz coconut rum
- 1 oz Pineapple juice
- 2 tbsp Lite 85 vanilla yogurt

Directions

1. blend ingredients together in blender with about 12 ice cubes.
2. This makes one pina' colada

Tuna Melt

Ingredients

- 2 Whole wheat english muffins - Cut in half
- 1 6.5 oz. can tuna in water - drained
- 3/4 Cup cole slaw mix
- 1-1/2 Tbs. Light Mayo

- 1 Tbs. Dijon Mustard
- 1 Tbs. Dill Weed - dried
- ! green onion sliced
- 1/3 C. Reduced fat cheddar cheese shreads
- Pepper to taste

Directions

1. Mix together Mayo, Dijon mustard and Dill Weed in med bowl.
2. Add drained tuna flaking it, cole slaw mix and green onion. Mix well.
3. Lightly toast english muffins. Place tuna mixture onto each half dividing it equally.
4. Top with cheddar cheese and broil 4 inches from element in oven or toaster oven for 3-4 minutes or until cheese is melted.

Egg & new potato salad

Prep: 5 mins - 10 mins, Easy

Nutrition: kcal: 0 fat: 0g saturates: 0g carbs: 0g sugars: 0g fibre: 0g protein: 0g low in salt: 0g

Ingredients

- hot boiled new potatoes
- 2 tbsp olive oil
- juice of 1/2 lemon
- handful chopped parsley
- hard-boiled egg

• bag of wild rocket

• cucumber, diced, to serve

Direction

1. Toss some hot boiled new potatoes with the olive oil, lemon juice and parsley. Leave to cool, then toss with quartered hard-boiled eggs. Toss with wild rocket leaves and some diced cucumber to serve.

Healthy fish & chips with tartare sauce

Prep: 5 mins Cook: 40 mins Ready in 40-45 mins, Easy, Serves: 2

Nutrition per serving: kcal: 373 fat: 9g saturates: 1g carbs: 41g sugars: 0g fibre: 3g protein: 35g low in salt: 0.96g

Ingredients

• 450g potatoes, peeled and cut into chips

- 1 tbsp olive oil, plus a little extra for brushing
- 2 white fish fillets about 140g/5oz each
- grated zest and juice 1 lemon
- small handful of parsley leaves, chopped
- 1 tbsp capers, chopped
- 2 heaped tbsp 0% Greek yogurt
- lemon wedge, to serve

Direction

1. Heat oven to 200C/fan 180C/gas 6. Toss chips in oil. Spread over a baking sheet in an even layer, bake for 40 mins until browned and crisp. Put the fish in a shallow dish, brush lightly with oil, salt and pepper. Sprinkle with half the lemon juice, bake for 12-15 mins. After 10 mins sprinkle over a little parsley and lemon zest to finish cooking.

2. Meanwhile, mix the capers, yogurt, remaining parsley and lemon juice together, set aside and season if you wish. To serve, divide the chips between plates, lift the fish onto the plates and serve with a spoonful of yogurt mix.

RECIPE TIPS: Swap the potatoes for sweet potatoes for a more exotic flavor. Or use turkey or skinless chicken fillets instead of fish if you prefer - simply bake 10 mins extra.

Perfect scrambled eggs recipe

Total time: 20 mins, Easy, Easily doubled

Nutrition: per serving (with milk): kcal: 254 fat: 19g saturates: 7g carbs: 4g sugars: 0g fibre: 0g protein: 18g low in salt: 0.6g

Ingredients

- 2 large free-range eggs
- 6 tbsp single cream or full cream milk

• a knob of butter

Direction

1. Lightly whisk 2 large eggs, 6 tbsp single cream or full cream milk and a pinch of salt together until the mixture has just one consistency.

2. Heat a small non-stick frying pan for a minute or so, then add a knob of butter and let it melt. Don't allow the butter to brown or it will discolour the eggs.

3. Pour in the egg mixture and let it sit, without stirring, for 20 seconds. Stir with a wooden spoon, lifting and folding it over from the bottom of the pan.

4. Let it sit for another 10 seconds then stir and fold again.

5. Repeat until the eggs are softly set and slightly runny in places. Remove from the heat and leave for a moment to finish cooking.

6. Give a final stir and serve the velvety scramble without delay.

Potato salad with anchovy & quail's eggs

Prep: 10 mins Cook: 20 mins Easy, Serves 1

This healthy, satisfying salad makes a tasty packed lunch or light supper with green beans, parsley, chives and lemon

Nutrition per serving: low in kcal: 174 low in fat: 5g saturates: 2g carbs: 20g sugars: 4g fibre: 5g protein: 9g salt: 0.5g

Ingredients

- 4 quail's eggs

- 100g green beans
- 100g new potatoes, halved or quartered if very large
- 1 anchovy, finely chopped
- 1 tbsp chopped parsley
- 1 tbsp chopped chives
- juice 0.5 lemon

Direction

1. Bring a medium pan of water to a simmer. Lower the quail's eggs into the water and cook for 2 mins. Lift out the eggs with a slotted spoon and put into a bowl of cold water. Add the beans to the pan, simmer for 4 mins until tender, then remove from the pan with a slotted spoon and plunge into the bowl of cold water.

2. Put the potatoes in the pan and boil for 10-15 mins until tender. Drain the potatoes in a colander and leave them to

cool. While the potatoes are cooling, peel the eggs and cut them in half. Toss the potatoes and beans with the chopped anchovy, herbs and lemon juice. Top with the quail's eggs to serve.

Gluten-free carrot cake

Prep: 20 mins Cook: 55 mins, Easy, Serves 8

Nutrition: kcal: 599 fat: 28g saturates: 16g carbs: 86g sugars: 64g fibre: 2g protein: 6g low in salt: 0.6g

Ingredients

- 140g unsalted butter, softened, plus extra for greasing
- 200g caster sugar
- 250g carrots, grated
- 140g sultanas
- 2 eggs, lightly beaten

- 200g gluten-free self-rising flour
- 1 tsp cinnamon
- 1 tsp gluten-free baking powder
- 50g mixed nut, chopped
- For the icing
- 75g butter, softened
- 175g icing sugar
- 3 tsp cinnamon, plus extra for dusting

Direction

1. Heat oven to 180C/160C fan/gas 4. Grease and line a 900g/2lb loaf tin with baking parchment.
2. Beat the butter and sugar until soft and creamy, then stir in the grated carrot and sultanas. Pour the eggs into the mix a little at a time.

3. Add the flour, cinnamon, baking powder and most of the chopped nuts and mix well. Tip the mix into the loaf tin, then bake for 50-55 mins or until a skewer poked in the middle comes out clean. Allow to cool in the tin for 15 mins, then remove from the tin and cool completely on a wire rack.

4. Meanwhile, make the icing. Beat the butter in a large bowl until it is really soft, add the icing sugar and cinnamon, then beat until thick and creamy. When the cake is cool, spread the icing on top, then sprinkle with a little more cinnamon and the remaining chopped nuts.

Pineapple & ginger Pavlova

Prep: 25 mins Cook :1 hr plus 8 hrs cooling, Serves 8

Nutrition: kcal: 493 fat: 34g saturates: 21g carbs: 44g sugars: 43g fibre: 1g protein: 3g salt: 0.1g

Ingredients

- 4 large egg whites
- 225g white caster sugar
- 1 tsp ground ginger
- 1 tsp cornflour
- 1 tsp white wine vinegar
- ½ large pineapple, peeled, cored and cut into 4-5 wedges
- 3 tbsp ginger syrup from the jar (see below), plus extra to drizzle
- 6 balls stem ginger in syrup, roughly chopped
- 500ml double cream
- 1 tbsp icing sugar, plus extra for dusting handful mint leaves, shredded

Direction

1. Heat oven to 150C/130C fan/gas 2. Place the egg whites in a large very clean bowl, and whisk to stiff peaks with an electric hand whisk. Continue to whisk while you add the sugar, 1 tbsp at a time, until the mixture is thick and glossy. Continue to whisk as you add the ginger, cornflour and vinegar.

2. Draw a 23cm circle on a piece of baking parchment, then turn it over and place on a large baking tray. Spread out the meringue mixture to fill the circle, creating a dip in the middle and higher sides. Run a palette knife up the edges at regular intervals if you want to create ridges. Bake for 1 hr, then leave in the oven with the door shut for 8 hrs until the Pavlova is completely cool.

3. While the Pavlova bakes, heat a clean griddle pan over a medium-high heat until hot. Brush the pineapple wedges with the ginger syrup and griddle for 2 mins until char lines appear and the pineapple is slightly softened. Leave to cool

completely, then cut into chunks. (The pineapple can be griddled the day before and chilled. Let it come to room temperature before you assemble the Pavlova. The Pavlova base can be made up to 2 days before serving, stored in an airtight container, then topped with cream and pineapple just before serving).

4. When you're ready to serve, whizz the stem ginger and 2 tbsp of the syrup in the small bowl of a food processor to a chunky paste. Add the cream and icing sugar and whip to soft peaks, then spoon into the crater of the meringue. Top with the pineapple, drizzle with a little extra ginger syrup, scatter over the mint and dust with icing sugar.

Chilli cornbread

Prep: 20 mins Cook: 30 mins, plus at least 2 hrs soaking, More effort, Serves 4 - 6

Ingredients

- 200g polenta or fine ground cornmeal
- 284ml pot buttermilk
- 25g butter
- 1 red chilli, deseeded and finely chopped
- 1 tsp baking powder (look for a gluten-free one)
- ¼ tsp bicarbonate of soda
- 50g frozen sweetcorn, defrosted
- 2 large eggs, beaten

Direction

1. Lightly toast the polenta in a dry frying pan for 3-4 mins, stirring to ensure even cooking, until the polenta has heated through, is fragrant and small patches are starting to turn golden brown. Take off the heat, tip half into a large bowl and

add the buttermilk. Stir well, cover and leave to soak for 2-3 hrs.

2. Melt the butter in a 25cm ovenproof frying pan (a cast-iron one is perfect) and heat oven to 220C/200C fan/gas 7. Stir the butter and the remaining ingredients, including the rest of the toasted polenta and 1/2 tsp salt, into the buttermilk and polenta mixture. (Don't wipe out the frying pan – the slick of butter will ensure the bread doesn't stick.)

3. Put the pan back on the heat and turn up the temperature. Pour the mixture into the pan – it should sizzle as it hits it, like a Yorkshire pudding. Put the whole pan in the oven and bake for 15-20 mins until golden brown and firm in the middle. Leave to cool a little, then serve cut into wedges.

Yorkshire puddings

Prep: 5 mins Cook: 25 mins, Easy, Makes 24 small or 8 large

The perfect vehicle for gravy and roasted goodies: the Yorkshire pudding - this version is gluten-free but never fear, you still get that characteristic puff and golden colour

Nutrition: per pud (8 large) kcal: 199 fat: 13g saturates: 2g carbs: 15g sugars: 1g fibre: 0g protein: 6g salt: 0.12g

Ingredients

- 140g gluten-free plain flour
- 50g corn flour
- 3 eggs
- 175ml semi-skimmed milk
- sunflower oil, for drizzling

Direction

1. Make up the batter mix. Tip the flours into a bowl with 1/2 tsp salt, make a well in the middle and crack the eggs into it. Whisk it together, then slowly add the milk, whisking all the

time until lump-free. Leave to stand until you are ready to cook.

2. Heat oven to 230C/210C fan/gas 8. Drizzle a little oil evenly into two 12-hole non-stick muffin tins and put into the oven to heat through.

3. Pour the batter into a jug, then remove the hot tins from the oven. Carefully and evenly pour the batter into the holes. Put the tins back in the oven and leave undisturbed for 20-25 mins until the puddings have puffed up and browned. Serve immediately.

Chocolate, cardamom & hazelnut torte

Prep: 30 mins Cook: 40 mins Easy, Serves 8

This rich, gluten-free torte has an irresistible chocolate & spice mix. An easy weekend treat or dinner party dessert you can make in advance

Nutrition: kcal: 473 fat: 37g saturates: 15g carbs: 24g sugars: 21g fibre: 4g protein: 10g salt: 0.4g

Ingredients

- 150g blanched hazelnuts
- 8 green cardamom pods
- 150g gluten-free dark chocolate
- 125g butter
- 6 eggs, separated
- 125g golden caster sugar
- 1 tbsp cocoa powder, plus extra for dusting
- crème fraîche, to serve

Direction

1. Toast the hazelnuts in a dry pan until golden, then leave to cool slightly and blitz to a fine consistency in a food processor.

Remove the cardamom seeds from their pods and grind using a pestle and mortar.

2. Heat oven to 160C/140C fan/gas 3. Grease and line the base of a 23cm spring-form cake tin. Use a microwave to melt the chocolate with the butter in 30-sec bursts until glossy and smooth. Leave to cool slightly.

3. Using an electric whisk, in a very clean bowl whisk the egg whites until they reach stiff peaks. Then, without cleaning the beaters, whisk the yolks with the sugar in a separate bowl until pale and voluminous.

4. Combine the chocolate with the egg yolk mixture, then incorporate the cocoa powder, a pinch of salt, the cardamom seeds and hazelnuts. Add a spoonful of egg white to the batter, stirring it through to loosen the mix, then fold in the rest, taking care to keep in as much air as possible. Gently pour into the tin and bake for 35 mins. Leave to cool in the

tin, then dust with cocoa powder and serve with crème fraîche.

Printed in Great Britain
by Amazon

60359787R00066